CKD STAGE 4 COOKBOOK FOR SENIORS

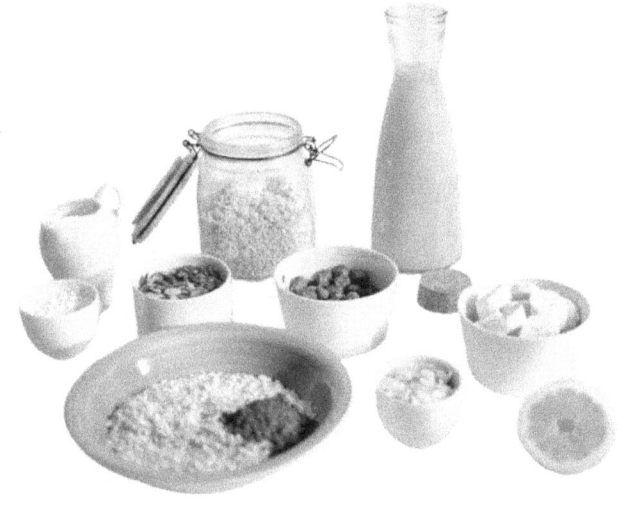

Creative Cooking for a CKD Stage 4 Diet for Seniors

Linda Carlucci

Copyright © 2024 by Linda Carlucci

DISCLAIMER

This cookbook is intended to provide general information and recipes.

The recipes provided in this cookbook are not intended to replace or be a substitute for medical advice from a physician.

The reader should consult a healthcare professional for any specific medical advice, diagnosis or treatment.

Any specific dietary advice provided in this cookbook is not intended to replace or be a substitute for medical advice from a physician.

The author is not responsible or liable for any adverse effects experienced by readers of this cookbook as a result of following the recipes or dietary advice provided.

The author makes no representations or warranties of any kind (express or implied) as to the accuracy, completeness, reliability or suitability of the recipes provided in this cookbook.

The author disclaims any and all liability for any damages arising out of the use or misuse of the recipes provided in this cookbook. The reader must also take care to ensure that the recipes provided in this cookbook are prepared and cooked safely.

The recipes provided in this cookbook are for informational purposes only and should not be used as a substitute for professional medical advice, diagnosis or treatment.

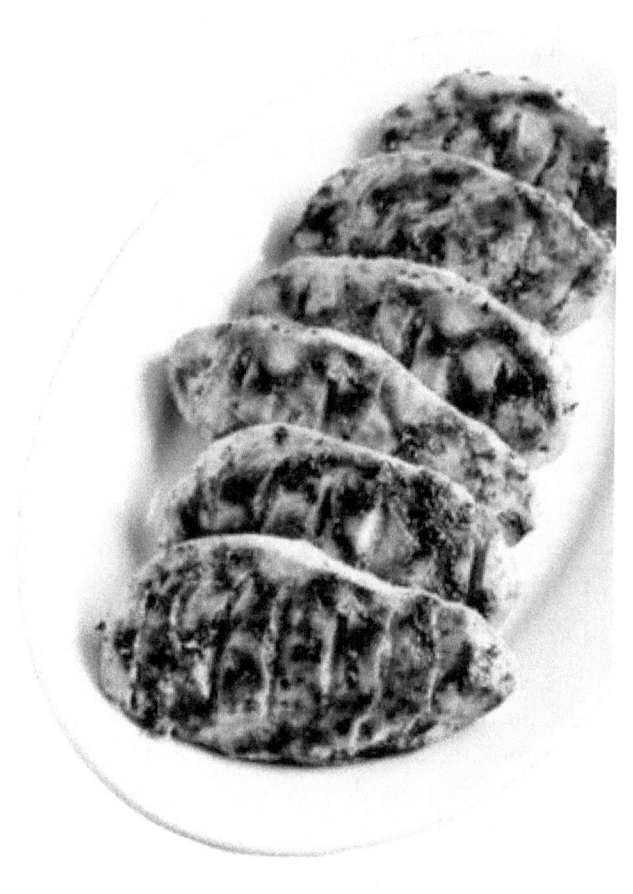

TABLE OF CONTENTS

INTRODUCTION

The illness known as chronic kidney disease (CKD) is characterized by a progressive decline in kidney function.

Because aging is a normal process that can cause a decline in kidney function, chronic kidney disease (CKD) can be especially difficult for seniors.

Seniors with CKD require a comprehensive approach that addresses their unique requirements and age-related changes.

Multiple health concerns, including high blood pressure, diabetes, and cardiovascular disease, are common in seniors with chronic kidney disease (CKD) and can exacerbate the condition. Consequently, to effectively control the symptoms of chronic kidney disease (CKD) and halt its progression, a comprehensive treatment plan is necessary.

An important factor in the management of CKD in elderly is diet. Seniors with CKD stage 3 diets should avoid meals heavy in potassium, phosphorus, salt, and protein since these might further tax the kidneys. Seniors are instead advised to consume foods low in these nutrients, such as lean protein sources like fish and chicken, fruits like apples and berries, and vegetables like cauliflower and cabbage.

Seniors with CKD may require medicine to control blood pressure, blood sugar, and cholesterol in addition to diet.

It is also critical to regularly check kidney function in order to spot any changes early and modify medication.

Maintaining a healthy lifestyle, which includes regular exercise, controlling weight, abstaining from tobacco and excessive alcohol use, is also crucial for seniors with chronic kidney disease (CKD).

Finally, you with CKD can manage your symptoms, decrease the disease's course, and enhance your overall quality of life by adhering to a thorough treatment plan.

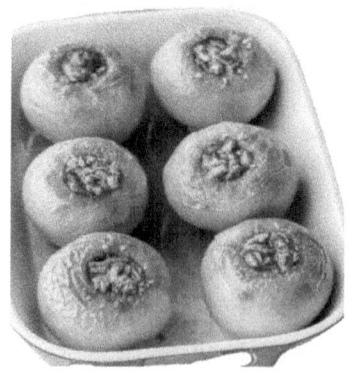

CHAPTER 1

SYMPTOMS OF CKD STAGE 4 IN SENIORS

1. Fatigue: Seniors with stage 4 CKD may feel weak and tired all the time, which can make it difficult for them to go about their everyday lives.

2. Fluid retention: Seniors may have swelling in their hands, faces, abdomens, or legs as a result of their kidneys' failure to adequately control fluid levels.

3. Shortness of breath: An accumulation of extra fluid in the lungs can make breathing difficult, particularly when one is lying down or exercising.

4. Nausea and vomiting: The body's accumulation of waste products can result in nausea and vomiting, which can impair appetite and induce weight loss.

5. Urinary pattern changes: Seniors with stage 4 CKD may notice changes in their frequency, color, or froth of their urine, as well as difficulties urinating.

6. High blood pressure: Chronic kidney disease (CKD) can cause high blood pressure, which raises the risk of heart disease and stroke as well as additional kidney damage.

7. Itching: Waste products can accumulate in the body and cause itching, especially on the skin.

8. Muscle cramps: Seniors with stage 4 CKD may have severe and disruptive muscle cramps, especially in the legs.

9. Sleep issues: Symptoms like itching, cramping in the muscles, or shortness of breath can make it difficult to go asleep or remain asleep.

10. Mental disorientation: Cognitive function abnormalities or mental disorientation may result from severe cases of CKD stage 4.

RISK FACTORS OF CKD STAGE 4

1. Diabetes: One of the main causes of CKD is diabetes. Over time, renal injury can result from high blood sugar levels damaging the blood vessels in the kidneys.

2. Hypertension (High Blood Pressure): High blood pressure can harm renal blood vessels and impair the kidneys' capacity to remove waste and fluid from the body, which can result in chronic kidney disease (CKD).

3. **Age:** CKD risk rises with age, particularly in the elderly. The structural and functional alterations brought on by aging kidneys may make it more difficult for them to filter waste.

4. **Obesity:** Being overweight raises the chance of getting chronic kidney disease (CKD) by altering hormone levels and raising the risk of other illnesses including diabetes and hypertension.

5. **Family History:** An increased risk of kidney disease, or CKD, can be attributed to a genetic predisposition if there is a history of the condition in one's family.

6. **Smoking:** Smoking raises the risk of chronic kidney disease (CKD) by damaging blood vessels and reducing blood flow to the kidneys.

7. **cardiovascular disease:** Because they can result in reduced blood flow to the kidneys, heart disease and stroke can raise the risk of chronic kidney disease (CKD).

8. High Cholesterol: By damaging the kidneys' blood arteries, high cholesterol can hasten the onset and course of chronic kidney disease (CKD).

9. Race or Ethnicity: People of African American, Native American, and Hispanic descent are among the racial and ethnic groups most at risk of having chronic kidney disease (CKD).

10. Other Chronic disorders: The chance of developing chronic kidney disease (CKD) is increased by disorders like kidney stones, urinary tract infections, and autoimmune diseases.

FOODS TO AVOID FOR CKD STAGE PATIENTS

1. High-Potassium Foods: Avoid consuming too much spinach, bananas, oranges, potatoes, tomatoes, and other foods high in potassium. High potassium levels can be dangerous for kidneys that are not working well since the kidneys cannot get rid of all the extra potassium in the blood.

2. High-Phosphorus Foods: You should restrict foods high in phosphorus, which include whole grains, dairy products, nuts, and seeds. CKD patients may have mineral and bone abnormalities as a result of high phosphorus levels.

3. High-salt Foods: You should restrict your intake of foods high in salt, such as processed meals, canned soups, and fast food. Consuming too much salt can cause blood pressure to rise and fluid retention, both of which can impair kidney function.

4. High-Protein Foods: Although protein is necessary for good health generally, consuming too much of it might strain the kidneys further. Meat, chicken, and fish are examples of high-protein foods that patients with stage 4 CKD should restrict their consumption of.

5. Processed meals: High amounts of salt, phosphorus, and other additives found in processed meals can be detrimental to kidney function. Processed food consumption should be restricted in patients with stage 4 CKD.

6. Foods High in Oxalates: You should restrict foods high in oxalates, like spinach, beets, and nuts. Kidney stones may develop as a result of elevated oxalate levels.

7. Carbonated Drinks: It is best to minimize your intake of carbonated drinks, such as soda and sparkling water. These drinks may contain a lot of phosphorus, which might lead to kidney stones.

8. Alcohol: Drinking too much alcohol might impair renal function; those with stage 4 CKD in particular should limit or stay away from it.

FOODS TO EAT

1. Low-Potassium Fruits: Fruits such as apples, berries, grapes, and pineapple are lower in potassium compared to bananas, oranges, and tomatoes. These fruits provide vitamins, minerals, and antioxidants without causing a significant increase in potassium levels.

2. Vegetables: Vegetables such as cauliflower, cabbage, bell peppers, and onions are lower in potassium and can be included in a kidney-friendly diet. These vegetables provide fiber, vitamins, and minerals without overloading the kidneys with potassium.

3. White Bread and Pasta: These are lower in phosphorus compared to whole grain options, making them a better choice for CKD stage 4

patients. However, portion control is important to avoid excessive calorie intake.

4. Lean Proteins: Lean protein sources such as chicken, fish, and eggs are recommended for CKD stage 4 patients. These proteins provide essential amino acids without overloading the kidneys with excess protein.

5. Low-Dairy or Dairy Alternatives: Dairy products are a good source of calcium and protein but can be high in phosphorus. Opting for lower phosphorus dairy options or dairy alternatives such as almond milk can help reduce phosphorus intake.

6. Oils and Fats: Healthy fats such as olive oil, avocado oil, and canola oil can be included in moderation. These fats provide essential fatty acids without negatively impacting kidney health.

7. Rice and Pasta: These are low in potassium and can be included in a kidney-friendly diet. However, portion control is important to avoid excessive calorie intake.

8. Applesauce and Cranberry Juice: These are lower in potassium and can be included in a kidney-friendly

diet. They also provide antioxidants and can help maintain hydration.

SALT SUBSTITUTES AND HEALTHY ALTERNATIVES

1. **Herbs and Spices:** Instead of salt, use herbs and spices to add flavor to your meals. Herbs like basil, thyme, rosemary, and spices like cumin, turmeric, and cinnamon can enhance the taste of your food without adding sodium.

2. **Lemon Juice or Vinegar:** Adding a splash of lemon juice or vinegar to your dishes can add acidity and flavor without the need for salt.

3. **Salt-Free Seasoning Blends:** Look for salt-free seasoning blends at the store or make your own at home using a variety of herbs and spices.

4. **Garlic and Onion:** Fresh or powdered garlic and onion can add flavor to your dishes without the need for salt.

5. **Low-Sodium Broth or Stock:** Use low-sodium broth or stock as a base for soups, stews, and sauces instead of regular broth or stock.

6. **Vegetables and Fruits:** Incorporate more vegetables and fruits into your diet, as they are naturally low in sodium and can add flavor and nutrients to your meals.

7. **Fresh or Frozen Foods:** Choose fresh or frozen foods over canned foods, as canned foods often contain added sodium for preservation.

8. **Read Food Labels:** When purchasing packaged or processed foods, read the labels and choose products that are low in sodium or salt-free.

BENEFITS OF A CKD DIET FOR SENIORS DEALING WITH STAGE 4 CKD

1. **Manage Symptoms:** A CKD diet can help manage symptoms such as fatigue, fluid retention, and high blood pressure, improving overall quality of life.

2. **Slow Disease Progression:** By reducing the intake of substances that can further damage the kidneys, a CKD diet can help slow the progression of the disease.

3. **Maintain Nutritional Balance:** A CKD diet is designed to provide adequate nutrition while limiting substances that can be harmful to the kidneys, helping seniors maintain a healthy diet.

4. **Prevent Complications:** By managing symptoms and slowing disease progression, a CKD diet can help prevent complications such as cardiovascular disease and mineral and bone disorders.

5. **Improve Overall Health:** A CKD diet that focuses on whole, nutrient-dense foods can improve overall health and well-being in seniors dealing with stage 4 CKD.

6. **Support Kidney Function:** By reducing the workload on the kidneys, a CKD diet can support kidney function and help preserve remaining kidney function.

7. **Reduce Medication Dependency:** A CKD diet that helps manage symptoms and slow disease progression may reduce the need for certain medications, improving quality of life.

CHAPTER 2

14-DAY MEAL PLAN

DAY 1

Breakfast: White Rice Milk and Cabbage Smoothie

Lunch: Cauliflower and Carrots Sauce on White Rice

Dinner: Roasted Vegetable with White Rice and Bell Peppers

DAY 2

Breakfast: Whole Grain Toast with Lettuce and Sliced Cucumber

Lunch: Grilled Vegetable Panini with Swiss Cheese

Dinner: Balsamic Marinated Zucchini

DAY 3

Breakfast: Fresh Raspberry and Cucumber Smoothie

Lunch: Egg White Salad Sandwich with Lettuce

Dinner: Wild Rice with Steamed Lettuce

DAY 4

Breakfast: Farina Porridge with Strawberries

Lunch: Cabbage Salad with Bell Peppers and Garlic

Dinner: Stuffed Bell Peppers with Shredded Chicken

DAY 5

Breakfast: White Bread Sandwich with Lettuce and Turkey

Lunch: Tofu and Cabbage Stir-Fry

Dinner: Lettuce Stuffed Skinless Chicken Breast

DAY 6

Breakfast: Swiss Cheese with Pear Slices

Lunch: Couscous Salad with Lemon Dressing

Dinner: Vegetarian Mexican Antojitos with Swiss Cheese

DAY 7

Breakfast: Egg White Scramble with Bell Peppers

Lunch: Wild Rice and Vegetable Stir-Fry

Dinner: Skinless Chicken and Cabbage Salad

DAY 8

Breakfast: Garlic Cauliflower Mash on White Bread Toast

Lunch: Carrot and Yellow Squash Wrap

Dinner: Spaghetti with Olive Oil, Garlic, and Parsley

DAY 9

Breakfast: Roasted Apple Salad

Lunch: Lemon Garlic Tilapia with Roasted Cauliflower

Dinner: Cucumber and Lettuce Sandwich

DAY1

Breakfast: Wild Rice Cinnamon Porridge with Stewed Apples

Lunch: Roasted Turkey Breast with Carrots and Green Beans

Dinner: Corn Tortilla with Sautéed Mushrooms and Lettuce

DAY 11

Breakfast: White Rice Milk and Cabbage Smoothie

Lunch: Cauliflower and Carrots Sauce on White Rice

Dinner: Roasted Vegetable with White Rice and Bell Peppers

DAY 12

Breakfast: Whole Grain Toast with Lettuce and Sliced Cucumber

Lunch: Grilled Vegetable Panini with Swiss Cheese

Dinner: Balsamic Marinated Zucchini

DAY 13

Breakfast: Fresh Raspberry and Cucumber Smoothie

Lunch: Egg White Salad Sandwich with Lettuce

Dinner: Wild Rice with Steamed Lettuce

DAY 14

Breakfast: Farina Porridge with Strawberries

Lunch: Cabbage Salad with Bell Peppers and Garlic

Dinner: Stuffed Bell Peppers with Shredded Chicken

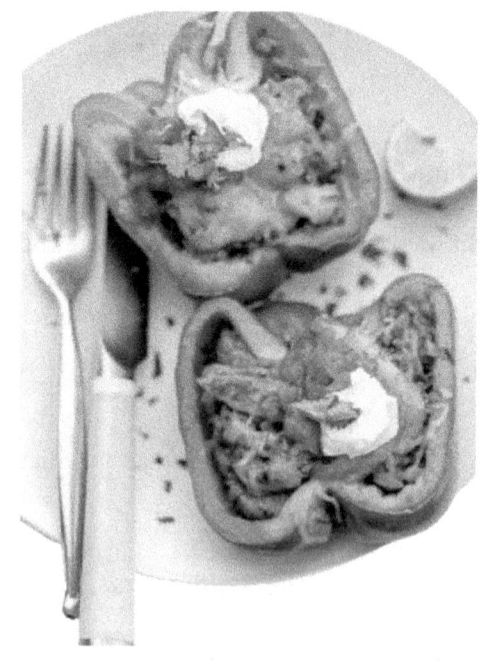

CHAPTER 3

NUTRITIOUS RECIPES FOR A CKD STAGE 4 DIET

BREAKFAST

White Rice Milk and Cabbage Smoothie

Preparation Time: 10 minutes

Serves: 2

Calories: 150 **Potassium:** 40mg **Phosphorus:** 50mg
Sugar: 4g

Ingredients:

1 cup cooked white rice

1 cup rice milk (unsweetened)

1 cup shredded cabbage

1/2 teaspoon ground cinnamon

1/4 teaspoon ground nutmeg

Ice cubes (optional)

Method of Preparation:

1. In a blender, combine cooked white rice, rice milk, shredded cabbage, honey (if using), ground cinnamon, and ground nutmeg.
2. Blend until smooth.
3. Add ice cubes if desired and blend again until well combined.
4. Pour into glasses and serve immediately.

Whole Grain Toast with Lettuce and Sliced Cucumber

Preparation Time: 5 minutes

Serves: 2

Calories: 180 **Potassium:** 50mg **Phosphorus:** 60mg **Sugar:** 2g

Ingredients:

4 slices whole grain bread (low sodium)

2 tablespoons olive oil

1 cup shredded lettuce

1 small cucumber, thinly sliced

Herbs and spices (such as oregano, basil, or thyme) to taste

Method of Preparation:

1. Toast the whole grain bread slices until golden brown.
2. Brush the toasted bread slices with olive oil.
3. Top each slice with shredded lettuce and thinly sliced cucumber.
4. Sprinkle with herbs and spices to taste.
5. Serve immediately.

Fresh Raspberry and Cucumber Smoothie

Preparation Time: 5 minutes

Serves: 2

Calories: 120 **Potassium:** 45mg **Phosphorus:** 40mg **Sugar:** 5g

Ingredients:

1 cup fresh raspberries

1 small cucumber, peeled and diced

1 cup rice milk (unsweetened)

1 tablespoon honey (optional)

1/2 teaspoon vanilla extract

Ice cubes (optional)

Method of Preparation:

1. In a blender, combine fresh raspberries, diced cucumber, rice milk, honey (if using), and vanilla extract.
2. Blend until smooth.
3. Add ice cubes if desired and blend again until well combined.
4. Pour into glasses and serve immediately.

Farina Porridge with Strawberries

Preparation Time: 10 minutes

Serves: 2

Calories: 150 **Potassium:** 40mg **Phosphorus:** 50mg **Sugar:** 8g

Ingredients:

1/4 cup farina

1 1/2 cups water

1/2 cup sliced strawberries

1 tablespoon honey (optional)

Method of Preparation:

1. In a saucepan, boil the water.
2. Slowly sprinkle in farina, stirring constantly.
3. Reduce heat to low and cook for 3-5 minutes, stirring occasionally, until thickened.
4. Remove from heat and let it cool slightly.
5. Serve topped with sliced strawberries and drizzle with honey if desired.

White Bread Sandwich with Lettuce and Turkey

Preparation Time: 5 minutes

Serves: 2

Calories: 250 **Potassium:** 45mg **Phosphorus:** 55mg **Sugar:** 2g

Ingredients:

4 slices low sodium white bread

4 oz cooked turkey breast, thinly sliced

1 cup shredded lettuce

1 tablespoon olive oil

1/2 teaspoon dried oregano

1/2 teaspoon dried basil

Method of Preparation:

1. Brush one side of each bread slice with olive oil.
2. On two bread slices, layer turkey slices and shredded lettuce.
3. Sprinkle with dried oregano and basil.
4. Top with the remaining bread slices, oiled side facing out.
5. Cut sandwiches in half and serve.

Swiss Cheese with Pear Slices

Preparation Time: 5 minutes

Serves: 2

Calories: 200 **Potassium:** 30mg **Phosphorus:** 40mg **Sugar:** 12g

Ingredients:

4 slices low sodium Swiss cheese

1 ripe pear, thinly sliced

1 tablespoon chopped walnuts (optional)

Method of Preparation:

1. Arrange Swiss cheese slices on a serving plate.
2. Place pear slices on top of the cheese.
3. Sprinkle with chopped walnuts if desired.
4. Serve immediately.

Egg White Scramble with Bell Peppers

Preparation Time: 15 minutes

Serves: 2

Calories: 70 **Potassium:** 90mg **Phosphorus:** 20mg **Sugar:** 2g

Ingredients:

4 egg whites

1/2 red bell pepper, diced

1/2 green bell pepper, diced

1/2 onion, diced

1/4 teaspoon garlic powder

1/4 teaspoon black pepper

1 teaspoon olive oil

Method of Preparation:

1. Heat olive oil in a non-stick skillet over medium heat.
2. Add diced bell peppers and onions to the skillet.
3. Sauté until softened, about 3-4 minutes.
4. In a bowl, whisk the egg whites with garlic powder and black pepper.

5. Pour the egg mixture into the skillet with the sautéed peppers and onions.

6. Cook, stirring occasionally, until the eggs are set, about 3-4 minutes.

7. Serve hot.

Garlic Cauliflower Mash on White Bread Toast

Preparation Time: 20 minutes

Serves: 2

Calories: 110 **Potassium:** 60mg **Phosphorus:** 40mg **Sugar:** 2g

Ingredients:

1/2 head cauliflower, chopped

2 cloves garlic, minced

1/4 teaspoon onion powder

1/4 teaspoon black pepper

4 slices low-sodium white bread

1 teaspoon olive oil

Method of Preparation:

1. Steam or boil cauliflower until tender, about 8-10 minutes.

2. In a blender or food processor, combine cooked cauliflower, minced garlic, onion powder, and black pepper.

3. Blend until smooth.

4. Toast white bread slices.

5. Spread the cauliflower mash onto the toasted bread slices.

6. Drizzle with olive oil.

7. Serve warm.

Roasted Apple Salad

Preparation Time: 25 minutes

Serves: 2

Calories: 150 **Potassium:** 40mg **Phosphorus:** 40mg **Sugar:** 14g

Ingredients:

2 apples, cored and sliced

2 cups mixed greens

2 tablespoons chopped walnuts

1 tablespoon olive oil

1/4 teaspoon cinnamon

Method of Preparation:

1. Preheat oven to 375°F (190°C).
2. Place sliced apples on a baking sheet lined with parchment paper.
3. Sprinkle with cinnamon.
4. Roast in the preheated oven for 15-20 minutes, until tender.
5. In a large bowl, toss mixed greens with olive oil.
6. Divide the greens onto two plates.
7. Top with roasted apples and chopped walnuts.
8. Serve immediately.

Wild Rice Cinnamon Porridge with Stewed Apples

Preparation Time: 60 minutes

Serves: 2

Calories: 200 **Potassium:** 100mg **Phosphorus:** 40mg **Sugar:** 12g

Ingredients:

1/2 cup wild rice, uncooked

2 cups water

2 apples, peeled, cored, and diced

1/2 teaspoon cinnamon

1/4 teaspoon nutmeg

1 tablespoon honey (optional)

Method of Preparation:

1. In a medium saucepan, bring water to a boil. Add wild rice, reduce heat to low, cover, and simmer for 45-50 minutes, until rice is tender and water is absorbed.

2. In another saucepan, combine diced apples, cinnamon, nutmeg, and honey (if using) with a splash of water. Cook over medium heat until apples are soft and slightly caramelized, about 10-12 minutes.

3. Divide the cooked wild rice into two bowls.

4. Top with stewed apples.

5. Serve warm.

LUNCH

Cauliflower and Carrots Sauce on White Rice

Preparation Time: 30 minutes

Serves: 2

Calories: 200 **Potassium:** 40mg **Phosphorus:** 50mg
Sugar: 2g

Ingredients:

1 cup cauliflower florets

1 cup sliced carrots

2 cups low potassium vegetable broth

1 teaspoon garlic powder

1 teaspoon onion powder

1/2 teaspoon dried thyme

1/2 teaspoon dried basil

1/4 teaspoon black pepper

2 cups cooked white rice

Method of Preparation:

1. In a saucepan, combine cauliflower florets, sliced carrots, and low potassium vegetable broth.
2. Bring to a boil, then reduce heat and simmer for 15-20 minutes or until vegetables are tender.
3. Using a blender or immersion blender, puree the cooked vegetables until smooth.
4. Return the pureed mixture to the saucepan.
5. Stir in garlic powder, onion powder, dried thyme, dried basil, and black pepper.
6. Simmer for an additional 5 minutes, stirring occasionally.
7. Serve the cauliflower and carrots sauce over cooked white rice.

Grilled Vegetable Panini with Swiss Cheese

Preparation Time: 20 minutes

Serves: 2

Calories: 250 **Potassium:** 45mg **Phosphorus:** 40mg **Sugar:** 4g

Ingredients:

1 zucchini, sliced

1 yellow squash, sliced

1 red bell pepper, sliced

1 onion, sliced

1 teaspoon dried oregano

1 teaspoon dried basil

4 slices low potassium whole grain bread

2 slices low sodium Swiss cheese

Method of Preparation:

1. Preheat a grill or grill pan over medium heat.
2. Toss zucchini, yellow squash, red bell pepper, and onion slices with dried oregano and dried basil.
3. Grill the vegetables for 3-4 minutes per side, or until tender and lightly charred.

4. Assemble the sandwiches by layering grilled vegetables and Swiss cheese between slices of whole grain bread.

5. Heat a panini press or grill pan over medium heat. Grill the sandwiches for 2-3 minutes on each side, or until the bread is crispy and the cheese is melted.

Egg White Salad Sandwich with Lettuce

Preparation Time: 15 minutes

Serves: 2

Calories: 180 **Potassium:** 30mg **Phosphorus:** 45mg **Sugar:** 2g

Ingredients:

4 hard-boiled egg whites, chopped

2 tablespoons low sodium mayonnaise

1 teaspoon Dijon mustard

1 stalk celery, finely chopped

1 green onion, thinly sliced

1/4 teaspoon dried dill

4 slices low potassium whole grain bread

Lettuce leaves, for serving

Method of Preparation:

1. In a bowl, combine chopped hard-boiled egg whites, low sodium mayonnaise, Dijon mustard, chopped celery, sliced green onion, and dried dill.
2. Mix until well combined.
3. Divide the egg white salad mixture between two slices of whole grain bread.
4. Top with lettuce leaves and another slice of bread to form sandwiches.

Cabbage Salad with Bell Peppers and Garlic

Preparation Time: 15 minutes

Serves: 2

Calories: 120 **Potassium:** 30mg **Phosphorus:** 25mg **Sugar:** 4g

Ingredients:

4 cups shredded cabbage

1 red bell pepper, thinly sliced

1 yellow bell pepper, thinly sliced

2 cloves garlic, minced

2 tablespoons olive oil

1 tablespoon fresh lemon juice

1 teaspoon dried oregano

1 teaspoon dried basil

Salt-free herb seasoning, to taste

Black pepper, to taste

Method of Preparation:

1. In a large bowl, combine the shredded cabbage, sliced bell peppers, and minced garlic.
2. In a small bowl, whisk together the olive oil, lemon juice, dried oregano, dried basil, salt-free herb seasoning, and black pepper.

3. Pour the dressing over the cabbage mixture and toss until well coated.

4. Refrigerate for at least 30 minutes before serving.

5. Serve chilled.

Tofu and Cabbage Stir-Fry

Preparation Time: 25 minutes

Serves: 2

Calories: 210 **Potassium:** 40mg **Phosphorus:** 35mg **Sugar:** 3g

Ingredients:

1 block (14 oz) firm tofu, drained and cubed

4 cups shredded cabbage

1 onion, thinly sliced

2 cloves garlic, minced

2 tablespoons low-sodium soy sauce

1 tablespoon sesame oil

1 teaspoon grated ginger

1 teaspoon cornstarch (mixed with 1 tablespoon water)

1 teaspoon sesame seeds (for garnish)

Chopped green onions (for garnish)

Method of Preparation:

1. Heat a large skillet over medium heat.
2. Add the cubed tofu and cook until golden brown on all sides.
3. Remove from skillet and set aside.
4. In the same skillet, add the shredded cabbage, sliced onion, and minced garlic.
5. Stir-fry for 3-4 minutes until the vegetables are tender-crisp.
6. In a small bowl, whisk together the low-sodium soy sauce, sesame oil, and grated ginger.
7. Return the tofu to the skillet.
8. Pour the sauce over the tofu and cabbage mixture.
9. Stir in the cornstarch mixture to thicken the sauce.
10. Cook for an additional 2-3 minutes until heated through.
11. Garnish with sesame seeds and chopped green onions before serving.

Couscous Salad with Lemon Dressing

Preparation Time: 15 minutes

Serves: 2

Calories: 280 **Potassium:** 50mg **Phosphorus:** 40mg
Sugar: 2g

Ingredients:

1 cup couscous

1 1/4 cups water

1/4 cup diced cucumber

1/4 cup diced bell pepper (any color except red)

1/4 cup diced red onion

2 tablespoons chopped fresh parsley

2 tablespoons olive oil

2 tablespoons fresh lemon juice

1 teaspoon lemon zest

1/2 teaspoon ground cumin

Salt-free herb seasoning, to taste

Black pepper, to taste

Method of Preparation:

1. In a medium saucepan, bring water to a boil.
2. Stir in couscous, cover, and remove from heat.
3. Let it sit for 5 minutes, then fluff with a fork and transfer to a large bowl to cool.
4. Once cooled, add diced cucumber, bell pepper, red onion, and chopped parsley to the couscous.
5. In a small bowl, whisk together the olive oil, fresh lemon juice, lemon zest, ground cumin, salt-free herb seasoning, and black pepper.
6. Pour the dressing over the couscous mixture and toss until well combined.
7. Refrigerate for at least 30 minutes before serving.
8. Serve chilled.

Wild Rice and Vegetable Stir-Fry

Preparation Time: 60 minutes

Serves: 2

Calories: 250 **Potassium:** 45mg **Phosphorus:** 50mg
Sugar: 3g

Ingredients:

1 cup wild rice

2 cups low-sodium vegetable broth

1 tablespoon olive oil

1 small onion, diced

2 cloves garlic, minced

1 cup carrots, thinly sliced

1 cup yellow squash, thinly sliced

1 cup broccoli florets

1 cup bell peppers, thinly sliced

2 tablespoons low-sodium soy sauce

1 teaspoon ginger, grated

1 teaspoon dried basil

1 teaspoon dried thyme

Freshly ground black pepper, to taste

Method of Preparation:

1. In a medium saucepan, bring the vegetable broth to a boil.

2. Add wild rice, reduce heat to low, cover, and simmer for 45 minutes or until rice is tender and liquid is absorbed.

3. In a large skillet, heat olive oil over medium heat.

4. Add diced onion and minced garlic, sauté until softened, about 2 minutes.

5. Add carrots, yellow squash, broccoli, and bell peppers to the skillet.

6. Cook for 5-7 minutes or until vegetables are tender-crisp.

7. Stir in cooked wild rice, soy sauce, grated ginger, dried basil, dried thyme, and black pepper.

8. Cook for an additional 2-3 minutes, stirring occasionally, until heated through.

9. Serve hot and enjoy!

Carrot and Yellow Squash Wrap

Preparation Time: 30 minutes

Serves: 2

Calories: 320 **Potassium:** 40mg **Phosphorus:** 60mg **Sugar:** 3g

Ingredients:

4 large whole wheat tortillas

2 medium carrots, shredded

1 medium yellow squash, thinly sliced

2 tablespoons olive oil

1 teaspoon dried thyme

1 teaspoon dried oregano

1 teaspoon garlic powder

1 teaspoon onion powder

Salt-free seasoning blend, to taste

Freshly ground black pepper, to taste

1 cup shredded lettuce

Method of Preparation:

1. Preheat the oven to 375°F (190°C).

2. In a large bowl, toss the shredded carrots and sliced yellow squash with olive oil, dried thyme, dried oregano, garlic powder, onion powder, salt-free seasoning blend, and black pepper.

3. Spread the seasoned carrots and squash on a baking sheet lined with parchment paper.

4. Roast in the preheated oven for 20-25 minutes, or until tender and slightly browned.

5. Warm the whole wheat tortillas according to package instructions.

6. To assemble the wraps, divide the roasted carrots and squash among the tortillas.

7. Top with shredded lettuce.

8. Roll up the tortillas tightly, slice in half, and serve.

Lemon Garlic Tilapia with Roasted Cauliflower

Preparation Time: 25 minutes

Serves: 2

Calories: 220 **Potassium:** 45mg **Phosphorus:** 50mg

Sugar: 2g

Ingredients:

2 tilapia fillets

1 lemon, juiced and zested

2 cloves garlic, minced

2 tablespoons olive oil

Salt-free seasoning blend, to taste

Freshly ground black pepper, to taste

1 head cauliflower, cut into florets

1 tablespoon chopped fresh parsley (optional)

Method of Preparation:

1. Preheat the oven to 400°F (200°C).
2. In a small bowl, whisk together the lemon juice, lemon zest, minced garlic, and olive oil.
3. Place the tilapia fillets on a baking sheet lined with parchment paper. Brush the lemon garlic mixture over the tilapia fillets. Season with salt-free seasoning blend and black pepper.

4. Arrange the cauliflower florets on another baking sheet. Drizzle with olive oil and season with salt-free seasoning blend and black pepper.

5. Roast the tilapia and cauliflower in the preheated oven for 15-20 minutes, or until the tilapia is cooked through and flakes easily with a fork, and the cauliflower is tender and golden brown.

6. Garnish the tilapia with chopped fresh parsley, if desired, before serving.

Cucumber and Lettuce Sandwich

Preparation Time: 10 minutes

Serves: 2

Calories: 180 **Potassium:** 30mg **Phosphorus:** 40mg **Sugar:** 2g

Ingredients:

4 slices whole wheat bread

1 cucumber, thinly sliced

2 cups shredded lettuce

1/4 cup hummus (low-sodium, if available)

1 tablespoon chopped fresh dill

1 tablespoon chopped fresh chives

Freshly ground black pepper, to taste

Method of Preparation:

1. Spread hummus evenly on each slice of whole wheat bread.

2. Layer cucumber slices and shredded lettuce on two slices of bread.

3. Sprinkle chopped fresh dill and chives over the cucumber and lettuce.

4. Season with freshly ground black pepper, to taste.

5. Top with the remaining slices of bread to form sandwiches.

6. Cut each sandwich in half, if desired, and serve.

Roasted Turkey Breast with Carrots and Green Beans

Preparation Time: 40 minutes

Serves: 2

Calories: 250 **Potassium:** 40mg **Phosphorus:** 80mg **Sugar:** 5g

Ingredients:

1 pound turkey breast, boneless and skinless

2 cups carrots, peeled and sliced

2 cups green beans, trimmed

1 tablespoon olive oil

1 teaspoon dried thyme

1 teaspoon dried rosemary

1 teaspoon garlic powder

1/2 teaspoon black pepper

Fresh parsley for garnish (optional)

Method of Preparation:

1. Preheat your oven to 375°F (190°C).
2. In a small bowl, mix together olive oil, dried thyme, dried rosemary, garlic powder, and black pepper.
3. Place the turkey breast in a baking dish and brush it with the herb and olive oil mixture.

4. Arrange the carrots and green beans around the turkey breast in the baking dish.

5. Roast in the preheated oven for 25-30 minutes, or until the turkey is cooked through and vegetables are tender.

6. Let the turkey rest for a few minutes before slicing.

7. Serve the roasted turkey breast with carrots and green beans, garnished with fresh parsley if desired.

Roasted Vegetable with White Rice and Bell Peppers

Preparation Time: 30 minutes

Serves: 2

Calories: 200 **Potassium:** 50mg **Phosphorus:** 60mg **Sugar:** 3g

Ingredients:

2 cups mixed vegetables (such as bell peppers, zucchini, and carrots), diced

1 tablespoon olive oil

1 teaspoon dried thyme

1 teaspoon dried oregano

1 teaspoon garlic powder

1/2 teaspoon black pepper

1 cup white rice, cooked

Method of Preparation:

1. Preheat your oven to 400°F (200°C).
2. In a large bowl, toss the mixed vegetables with olive oil, dried thyme, dried oregano, garlic powder, and black pepper until evenly coated.
3. Spread the seasoned vegetables in a single layer on a baking sheet.
4. Roast in the preheated oven for 20-25 minutes, or until the vegetables are tender and slightly browned.
5. Serve the roasted vegetables with cooked white rice.

Balsamic Marinated Zucchini

Preparation Time: 35 minutes (including marinating time)

Serves: 2

Calories: 100 **Potassium:** 30mg **Phosphorus:** 40mg **Sugar:** 5g

Ingredients:

2 medium zucchinis, sliced

1 tablespoon olive oil

1 teaspoon dried basil

1 teaspoon dried oregano

1 teaspoon garlic powder

1/2 teaspoon black pepper

Method of Preparation:

1. In a small bowl, whisk together olive oil, dried basil, dried oregano, garlic powder, and black pepper.
2. Place the sliced zucchinis in a shallow dish and pour the balsamic marinade over them.
3. Toss to coat evenly.
4. Cover and refrigerate for at least 30 minutes to allow the flavors to meld.
5. Heat a grill pan or skillet over medium heat.
6. Add the marinated zucchini slices and cook for 3-4 minutes on each side, or until tender and lightly charred.

7. Serve the balsamic marinated zucchini as a side dish.

Wild Rice with Steamed Lettuce

Preparation Time: 60 minutes

Serves: 2

Calories: 250 **Potassium:** 40mg **Phosphorus:** 50mg **Sugar:** 1g

Ingredients:

1 cup wild rice

2 cups low sodium vegetable broth

2 cups shredded lettuce

1 tablespoon olive oil

1 teaspoon dried thyme

1 teaspoon dried parsley

1/4 teaspoon black pepper

Method of Preparation:

1. Rinse the wild rice under cold water.

2. In a medium saucepan, bring the vegetable broth to a boil.

3. Add the wild rice to the boiling broth, then reduce heat to low, cover, and simmer for 45-50 minutes or until rice is tender and liquid is absorbed.

4. While the rice is cooking, heat olive oil in a skillet over medium heat.

5. Add the shredded lettuce to the skillet and sauté for 3-4 minutes until wilted.

6. Once the rice is cooked, fluff it with a fork and transfer it to a serving dish.

7. Stir in the sautéed lettuce, dried thyme, dried parsley, and black pepper.

8. Serve warm.

Stuffed Bell Peppers with Shredded Chicken

Preparation Time: 45 minutes

Serves: 2

Calories: 220 **Potassium:** 45mg **Phosphorus:** 40mg **Sugar:** 2g

Ingredients:

2 large bell peppers (any color)

1 cup cooked and shredded chicken breast

1/2 cup cooked couscous

1/4 cup diced onion

1/4 cup diced celery

1/4 teaspoon garlic powder

1/4 teaspoon dried oregano

1/4 teaspoon dried basil

1/4 teaspoon black pepper

Method of Preparation:

1. Preheat the oven to 375°F (190°C).
2. Cut the tops off the bell peppers and remove the seeds and membranes.
3. In a mixing bowl, combine the shredded chicken, cooked couscous, diced onion, diced celery, garlic powder, dried oregano, dried basil, and black pepper.
4. Stuff the mixture evenly into the bell peppers.

5. Place the stuffed bell peppers in a baking dish and cover with foil.

6. Bake for 25-30 minutes or until the peppers are tender.

7. Remove from the oven and let cool for a few minutes before serving.

Lettuce Stuffed Skinless Chicken Breast

Preparation Time: 40 minutes

Serves: 2

Calories: 230 **Potassium:** 50mg **Phosphorus:** 45mg **Sugar:** 1g

Ingredients:

2 skinless, boneless chicken breasts

2 cups shredded lettuce

1/4 cup diced onion

1/4 cup diced bell pepper (any color)

1/4 teaspoon garlic powder

1/4 teaspoon dried thyme

1/4 teaspoon paprika

1 tablespoon olive oil

Method of Preparation:

1. Preheat the oven to 375°F (190°C).
2. In a skillet, heat olive oil over medium heat.
3. Add diced onion and bell pepper to the skillet and sauté until softened, about 3-4 minutes.
4. Add shredded lettuce to the skillet and cook for an additional 2-3 minutes until wilted.
5. Remove from heat and let cool slightly.
6. Butterfly each chicken breast by slicing horizontally, being careful not to cut all the way through.
7. Open up each chicken breast and place a portion of the cooked lettuce mixture inside.
8. Close the chicken breasts and secure with toothpicks if necessary.
9. Season the outside of the chicken breasts with garlic powder, dried thyme, and paprika.
10. Place the stuffed chicken breasts in a baking dish and bake for 25-30 minutes or until cooked through.

11. Serve warm.

Vegetarian Mexican Antojitos with Swiss Cheese

Preparation Time: 20 minutes

Serves: 2

Calories: 200 **Potassium:** 40mg **Phosphorus:** 50mg **Sugar:** 1g

Ingredients:

6 small corn tortillas

1/2 cup canned black beans, drained and rinsed (low sodium)

1/2 cup shredded low-sodium Swiss cheese

1/4 cup diced red bell pepper

1/4 cup diced green bell pepper

1/4 cup diced onion

1/2 teaspoon ground cumin

1/2 teaspoon chili powder

1/4 teaspoon garlic powder

1/4 teaspoon paprika

Cooking spray

Method of Preparation:

1. Preheat the oven to 375°F (190°C).
2. In a small bowl, mix together the black beans, diced bell peppers, onion, cumin, chili powder, garlic powder, and paprika.
3. Place the corn tortillas on a baking sheet lined with parchment paper. Spoon the bean mixture evenly onto each tortilla.
4. Sprinkle shredded Swiss cheese over the bean mixture on each tortilla.
5. Bake in the preheated oven for 8-10 minutes, or until the cheese is melted and the edges of the tortillas are crispy.
6. Remove from the oven and let cool slightly before Serving.

Skinless Chicken and Cabbage Salad

Preparation Time: 25 minutes

Serves: 2

Calories: 250 **Potassium:** 45mg **Phosphorus:** 40mg **Sugar:** 2g

Ingredients:

2 skinless, boneless chicken breasts

4 cups shredded green cabbage

1/4 cup chopped fresh cilantro

2 tablespoons chopped green onions

1 tablespoon olive oil

1/2 teaspoon ground cumin

1/2 teaspoon paprika

1/4 teaspoon garlic powder

1/4 teaspoon black pepper

Method of Preparation:

1. Season the chicken breasts with ground cumin, paprika, garlic powder, and black pepper.
2. Heat olive oil in a skillet over medium heat.
3. Cook the seasoned chicken breasts for 6-8 minutes on each side, or until cooked through.

4. Remove from the skillet and let cool slightly.

5. Slice the cooked chicken breasts into thin strips.

6. In a large bowl, combine the shredded cabbage, chopped cilantro, chopped green onions, and cooked chicken strips.

7. Toss until well mixed.

8. Divide the salad between two plates and serve immediately.

Spaghetti with Olive Oil, Garlic, and Parsley

Preparation Time: 20 minutes

Serves: 2

Calories: 300 **Potassium:** 40mg **Phosphorus:** 100mg **Sugar:** 1g

Ingredients:

200g whole grain spaghetti

2 tablespoons olive oil

3 cloves garlic, minced

2 tablespoons fresh parsley, chopped

1/4 teaspoon black pepper

1/4 teaspoon dried basil

1/4 teaspoon dried oregano

1/4 teaspoon dried thyme

1/4 teaspoon dried rosemary

Method of Preparation:

1. Cook the spaghetti according to package instructions.
2. Drain and set aside.
3. In a large skillet, heat olive oil over medium heat. Add minced garlic and sauté until fragrant, about 1-2 minutes.
4. Add cooked spaghetti to the skillet with garlic.
5. Sprinkle with black pepper, dried basil, dried oregano, dried thyme, and dried rosemary. Toss well to coat.
6. Remove from heat and stir in chopped parsley.
7. Serve hot.

Corn Tortilla with Sautéed Mushrooms and Lettuce

Preparation Time: 15 minutes

Serves: 2

Calories: 180 **Potassium:** 45mg **Phosphorus:** 70mg **Sugar:** 1g

Ingredients:

4 corn tortillas

1 cup sliced mushrooms

1 tablespoon olive oil

1/4 teaspoon garlic powder

1/4 teaspoon onion powder

1/4 teaspoon paprika

1/4 teaspoon black pepper

2 cups shredded lettuce

Method of Preparation:

1. Heat olive oil in a skillet over medium heat.

2. Add sliced mushrooms and sauté until tender, about 5 minutes.

3. Sprinkle garlic powder, onion powder, paprika, and black pepper over the mushrooms.

4. Stir well to coat evenly.

5. Warm corn tortillas in a separate skillet or in the microwave.

6. Divide the sautéed mushrooms evenly among the warm corn tortillas.

7. Top each tortilla with shredded lettuce.

8. Fold the tortillas in half and serve immediately.

POULTRY MAINS

Grilled Chicken Breast with Lemon and Herbs

Preparation Time: 40 minutes

Serves: 2

Calories: 180 **Potassium:** 45mg **Phosphorus:** 120mg **Sugar:** 0g

Ingredients:

2 boneless, skinless chicken breasts

1 lemon, juiced and zested

1 tablespoon olive oil

1 teaspoon dried thyme

1 teaspoon dried rosemary

1 teaspoon dried oregano

Salt-free herb seasoning, to taste

Method of Preparation:

1. In a bowl, mix lemon juice, lemon zest, olive oil, thyme, rosemary, oregano, and salt-free herb seasoning.
2. Add chicken breasts to the marinade, making sure they are evenly coated.
3. Marinate in the refrigerator for at least 30 minutes.
4. Preheat grill to medium-high heat. Grill chicken breasts for 6-8 minutes per side, or until cooked through.
5. Serve hot with a wedge of lemon for garnish.

Baked Turkey Breast with Cranberry Sauce

Preparation Time: 40 minutes

Serves: 2

Calories: 220 **Potassium:** 35mg **Phosphorus:** 110mg **Sugar:** 6g

Ingredients:

1 turkey breast (about 1 pound)

1/4 cup unsweetened cranberry juice

1 tablespoon honey

1 teaspoon grated ginger

1/2 teaspoon ground cinnamon

1/4 teaspoon ground cloves

Method of Preparation:

1. Preheat oven to 350°F (175°C).
2. In a small saucepan, combine cranberry juice, honey, ginger, cinnamon, and cloves.

3. Cook over medium heat until the mixture thickens slightly, about 5 minutes.

4. Set aside.

5. Place the turkey breast in a baking dish and brush with half of the cranberry sauce.

6. Bake for 25-30 minutes, or until the turkey is cooked through, basting occasionally with the remaining cranberry sauce.

7. Let the turkey rest for a few minutes before slicing. Serve with extra cranberry sauce on the side.

Chicken Curry with White Rice Milk

Preparation Time: 45 minutes

Serves: 2

Calories: 230 **Potassium:** 40mg **Phosphorus:** 100mg **Sugar:** 1g

Ingredients:

2 boneless, skinless chicken breasts, cubed

1 onion, finely chopped

2 cloves garlic, minced

1 teaspoon grated ginger

1 tablespoon olive oil

1 teaspoon ground turmeric

1 teaspoon ground cumin

1 teaspoon ground coriander

1/2 teaspoon ground cinnamon

1/4 teaspoon ground cloves

1 cup unsweetened white rice milk

Salt-free curry powder, to taste

Method of Preparation:

1. Heat olive oil in a skillet over medium heat.
2. Add onion, garlic, and ginger.
3. Cook until softened, about 5 minutes.
4. Add cubed chicken breasts to the skillet.
5. Cook until browned on all sides, about 6-8 minutes.
6. Stir in turmeric, cumin, coriander, cinnamon, cloves, and salt-free curry powder.
7. Cook for another 2 minutes.

8. Pour in white rice milk and bring to a simmer. Reduce heat and let the curry simmer for 15-20 minutes, stirring occasionally, until the chicken is cooked through and the sauce has thickened.
9. Serve hot with steamed white rice.

Turkey Meatballs in Bell Pepper and Cabbage Sauce

Preparation Time: 40 minutes

Serves: 2

Calories: 320 **Potassium:** 40mg **Phosphorus:** 110mg **Sugar:** 3g

Ingredients:

1 lb. lean ground turkey

1/4 cup almond flour

1/4 cup chopped onion

1 clove garlic, minced

1/2 teaspoon dried oregano

1/2 teaspoon dried basil

1/4 teaspoon dried thyme

1/4 teaspoon black pepper

2 cups shredded cabbage

1 red bell pepper, thinly sliced

1 yellow bell pepper, thinly sliced

2 cups low-sodium chicken broth

1 tablespoon olive oil

Fresh parsley, for garnish

Method of Preparation:

1. Preheat the oven to 375°F (190°C).
2. In a large bowl, combine the ground turkey, almond flour, chopped onion, minced garlic, dried oregano, dried basil, dried thyme, and black pepper.
3. Mix until well combined, then shape into meatballs.
4. Heat the olive oil in a large skillet over medium heat.
5. Add the meatballs and cook until browned on all sides, about 5 minutes.
6. Add the shredded cabbage and sliced bell peppers to the skillet.

7. Cook for an additional 3 minutes.

8. Pour the chicken broth into the skillet and bring to a simmer.

9. Cover and transfer to the preheated oven.

10. Bake for 20 minutes, or until the meatballs are cooked through.

11. Serve the turkey meatballs with the bell pepper and cabbage sauce, garnished with fresh parsley.

Lemon Herb Roasted Chicken Thighs

Preparation Time: 35 minutes

Serves: 2

Calories: 280**Potassium:** 45mg **Phosphorus:** 150mg **Sugar:** 0g

Ingredients:

4 bone-in, skinless chicken thighs

1 tablespoon olive oil

2 cloves garlic, minced

1 teaspoon dried thyme

1 teaspoon dried rosemary

1 teaspoon dried parsley

1 lemon, thinly sliced

Fresh parsley, for garnish

Method of Preparation:

1. Preheat the oven to 400°F (200°C).
2. In a small bowl, combine the olive oil, minced garlic, dried thyme, dried rosemary, and dried parsley.
3. Place the chicken thighs in a baking dish.
4. Rub the herb mixture over the chicken thighs.
5. Arrange the lemon slices on top of the chicken thighs.
6. Roast in the preheated oven for 25-30 minutes, or until the chicken is cooked through and juices run clear.
7. Garnish with fresh parsley before serving.

SEAFOOD MAINS

Grilled Salmon with Lemon and Dill

Preparation Time: 20 minutes

Serves: 2

Calories: 250 **Potassium:** 40mg **Phosphorus:** 150mg **Sugar:** 0g

Ingredients:

2 salmon fillets (4-6 ounces each)

1 tablespoon olive oil

1 lemon, thinly sliced

2 teaspoons fresh dill, chopped

Salt-free herb seasoning, to taste

Method of Preparation:

1. Preheat grill to medium heat.
2. Brush both sides of the salmon fillets with olive oil and sprinkle with salt-free herb seasoning.
3. Place lemon slices on top of each fillet and sprinkle with fresh dill.
4. Grill salmon for 4-5 minutes on each side, or until cooked through.
5. Serve hot with additional lemon slices if desired.

Shrimp Scampi with Garlic and Herbs

Preparation Time: 15 minutes

Serves: 2

Calories: 180 **Potassium:** 30mg **Phosphorus:** 100mg **Sugar:** 0g

Ingredients:

12 large shrimp, peeled and deveined

2 tablespoons olive oil

4 cloves garlic, minced

2 tablespoons fresh parsley, chopped

1 tablespoon fresh basil, chopped

1 tablespoon fresh chives, chopped

Salt-free herb seasoning, to taste

Method of Preparation:

1. Heat olive oil in a skillet over medium heat.

2. Add minced garlic and cook until fragrant, about 1 minute.

3. Add shrimp to the skillet and cook for 2-3 minutes on each side, until pink and cooked through.

4. Stir in chopped parsley, basil, and chives. Season with salt-free herb seasoning to taste.

5. Serve hot, garnished with additional chopped herbs if desired.

Baked Cod with Lemon and Herbs

Preparation Time: 25 minutes

Serves: 2

Calories: 200 **Potassium:** 45mg **Phosphorus:** 120mg **Sugar:** 0g

Ingredients:

2 cod fillets (4-6 ounces each)

1 tablespoon olive oil

1 lemon, juiced

2 teaspoons fresh thyme, chopped

2 teaspoons fresh rosemary, chopped

Salt-free herb seasoning, to taste

Method of Preparation:

1. Preheat oven to 375°F (190°C).
2. Brush both sides of the cod fillets with olive oil and place them in a baking dish.
3. Drizzle lemon juice over the fillets and sprinkle with fresh thyme, rosemary, and salt-free herb seasoning.
4. Bake for 15-20 minutes, or until the fish is opaque and flakes easily with a fork.
5. Serve hot, with additional lemon wedges if desired.

Tuna Steak with Ginger Marinade

Preparation Time: 40 minutes (including marinating time)

Serves: 2

Calories: 250 **Potassium:** 45mg **Phosphorus:** 70mg
Sugar: 0g

Ingredients:

2 tuna steaks (about 6 ounces each)

2 tablespoons low-sodium soy sauce

2 tablespoons fresh lemon juice

1 tablespoon grated ginger

2 cloves garlic, minced

1 tablespoon olive oil

1/2 teaspoon ground black pepper

1 teaspoon dried parsley (or other herbs of choice)

Non-stick cooking spray

Method of Preparation:

1. In a small bowl, mix together the soy sauce, lemon juice, grated ginger, minced garlic, olive oil, black pepper, and dried parsley.

2. Place the tuna steaks in a shallow dish and pour the marinade over them, ensuring they are evenly coated. Cover and refrigerate for at least 30 minutes, or up to 2 hours.

3. Preheat a grill or grill pan over medium-high heat and lightly coat with non-stick cooking spray.

4. Remove the tuna steaks from the marinade and discard the excess marinade.

5. Grill the tuna steaks for 3-4 minutes per side, or until desired doneness.

6. Serve hot with a side of steamed vegetables or a green salad.

Grilled Shrimp Skewers with Vegetables

Preparation Time: 30 minutes

Serves: 2

Calories: 180 **Potassium:** 35mg **Phosphorus:** 60mg **Sugar:** 2g

Ingredients:

12 large shrimp, peeled and deveined

1 zucchini, sliced into rounds

1 yellow bell pepper, cut into chunks

1 red onion, cut into chunks

2 tablespoons olive oil

2 cloves garlic, minced

1 teaspoon dried Italian herb (basil, oregano, thyme)

1/2 teaspoon paprika

1/4 teaspoon ground black pepper

Bamboo skewers, soaked in water for 30 minutes

Method of Preparation:

1. In a small bowl, mix together the olive oil, minced garlic, Italian herbs, paprika, and black pepper.
2. Thread the shrimp, zucchini rounds, yellow bell pepper chunks, and red onion chunks onto the soaked bamboo skewers, alternating as desired.
3. Brush the skewers with the olive oil mixture, ensuring they are evenly coated.
4. Preheat a grill or grill pan over medium-high heat.
5. Grill the skewers for 2-3 minutes per side, or until the shrimp are pink and opaque.
6. Serve hot with a side of quinoa or brown rice.

CONCLUSION

In summary, stage 4 chronic kidney disease (CKD) affects seniors more than any other group and is a dangerous condition that needs to be carefully managed.

In order to control symptoms, decrease the progression of the illness, and enhance general health and well-being, a CKD diet is essential.

You can maintain a healthy diet while supporting renal function by adhering to a CKD diet that emphasizes foods that are high in nutrients, low in sodium, and low in phosphorus.

Reducing sodium intake is also possible with healthy alternatives and salt substitutes, which is crucial for blood pressure management and avoiding fluid retention.

Seniors can enhance flavor without using salt by adding herbs, spices, lemon juice, and other flavorings to their food.

If you have stage 4 CKD, you can benefit from a CKD diet in a number of ways, including as symptom management, disease progression slowing, and complication avoidance.

It can also support weight control and lessen reliance on prescription drugs.

You should collaborate closely with our healthcare professional or dietitian to create a customized food plan that satisfies your nutritional requirements and promotes kidney function if you have stage 4 CKD.